HERBS ESSENTIAL OILS FOR KILLING LYME, BABESIA, AND BARTONELLA

James L. Schaller, MD, MAR

Kimberly Mountjoy, MS

Copyright © 2023 by James Schaller, MD, MAR and Kimberly Mountjoy, MS

All rights reserved.

International Infectious Disease Press
Bank Tower • Newgate Center (Suite 305)
5150 Tamiami Trail North [Highway 41]
Naples, Florida 34103

To Kimberly Mountjoy, MS
Amazing Scientist,
Constantly Kind,
Profound Christian

Acknowledgment
Stephen H. Buhner
Thank you for everything

CONTENTS

Why Use Natural Treatments for Lyme Disease, *Babesia*, and *Bartonella*? 1

Why Promote These Herbal Options? 5

Sample Lyme, *Babesia*, and *Bartonella* Herbal Treatments 7

Herbs that Kill All Three—Lyme, *Babesia*, and *Bartonella* 9

The Good News 11

Cryptolepis sanguinolenta 13

Japanese Knotweed (*Polygonum cuspidatum*) 15

Andrographis (*Andrographis paniculata*) 17

Houttuynia cordata 21

Cat's Claw (Samento or *Uncaria tomentosa*) 23

Otoba parvifolia (Banderol) 25

Artemisia, Artesunate and Artemisinin 27

IV or Muscle-Injected Artesunate 31

Garlic and Synthetic Garlic 35

Black Walnut (*Juglans nigra*) 39

Alchornea cordifolia 41
Essential Oils Used Against Lyme, *Babesia*, and *Bartonella* 43
Chinese skullcap (*Scutellaria baicalensis* or Calvaria) 49
Cistus incanus (or *Cistus creticus*) 51
Teasel 53
Lowering "Herx" Reactions with Herbs 55
Chlorella 57
Dandelion Root 59
Modified Citrus Pectin 61
Optifiber Lean 63
Japanese Knotweed 65
Cannabis Derivatives 67
Quercetin 69

Endnotes 71
Bibliography 85

Why Use Natural Treatments for Lyme Disease, Babesia, and Bartonella?

First, these can be very brutal infections that can cause severe misery and hinder your functioning. So having every option is wise.

These infections have persister cells which survive after routine synthetic antibiotics. In the case of Lyme disease, the usual spiral-shaped bacteria can transform to have protective round bodies that resist prescription medications.

Most infections, such as Lyme and *Bartonella,* live behind a slimy biofilm that typical antibiotics struggle to penetrate. And according to a *Babesia* expert and friend, Dr. Henry Lindner, *Babesia* also lives in "nests" making it hard to see in routine blood tests.

Synthetic antibiotics consist of only one precise chemical which makes it easier for the bacteria to defeat the antibiotic. This is what we call "resistance." But herbs tend to have more than one killing agent. And it is hard to defeat multiple herbal antibiotics at the same time—each may have 1-3 antibiotic chemicals—that is a great deal of healing power.

For example, *Uncaria tomentosa* (Cat's Claw), at a very low concentration, showed profound reduction of Lyme's biofilm—the slimy layer that makes antibiotics fail, because they cannot penetrate the biofilms. But *Uncaria* does not kill the Lyme bacteria. However, adding *Otoba parvifolia* (Banderol) extract kills over 90 percent of the bacteria, while it had no effect on biofilms. Simply, let me share a critical truth up front. The treatment of Lyme, *Babesia*, and *Bartonella* requires different unique treatments, and if you are using herbs or synthetic drugs **you will always need more than one treatment**. You need medical combination treatment to have success.

If you look at naturopathic doctor (ND) herbal products, notice they usually have multiple agents in a liquid tincture or capsule.

One limitation of herbal and essential oil treatment is that the research on their use is limited. And most of the main studies on the use of herbs as bacteria killers are merely test-tube findings in a lab. There is little testing in humans or even mice. But they have all been used for hundreds, or even thousands, of years. I have prescribed them for 29 years to help heal my children, wife, patients, friends, and myself. Most advanced physicians routinely use synthetic medicines which have limited research for a particular illness. For example, Monica Embers published the effect of common and emerging synthetic drugs against *Bartonella* in the lab—not in humans or even rats or mice.[1] Useful lessons, but it is limited. Therefore, both natural and traditional medicine often need human trials to confirm findings in the test tube.

Why Promote These Herbal Options?

Simply, I am not writing a fat textbook about herbs and essential oils. This will be short and only give the bottom line or few readers will finish it. And many proposed herbal treatments for Lyme, *Babesia*, and *Bartonella* have minimal publications. So, this small book fills a need.

As a trend, herbal treatments have modest to low side effects, though not all are recommended during pregnancy. If you are pregnant or trying to conceive, consult a naturopathic doctor about any herb before use.

Since these tick or flea infections can be hard to cure fully, healers need every treatment option that makes sense.

Please note, most herbs have a common simple name and a technical name. I include this professional name because some books, stores, and research papers use the technical one.

I will only discuss the best natural options, so the list of herbs to learn will be small. And with this book open, you can easily order these yourself. Having the guidance of a Herbal Lyme expert or a naturopathic doctor might make purchasing easier. So, a herb may be listed as Japanese knotweed, or *Polygonum cuspidatum*. I will use both.

Sample Lyme, Babesia, and Bartonella Herbal Treatments

Feng and Zhang showed in a test-tube study that some natural treatments have a good ability to kill Lyme—possibly superior to doxycycline and cefuroxime (IV Rocephin).[2] Indeed, these researchers found that seven herbal extracts at only 1% potency killed Lyme effectively. These potent treatments were:

Polygonum cuspidatum root (Japanese knotweed)

Uncaria tomentosa (Cat's Claw or Samento)

Cryptolepis sanguinolenta

Scutellaria baicalensis (Chinese skullcap)

Artemisia annua (Sweet wormwood)

Juglans nigra (Black walnut)

Zhang found five herbs that interfere with *Babesia*.[3] These are:

> *Cryptolepis sanguinolenta*
>
> *Artemisia annua* (Sweet wormwood)
>
> *Scutellaria baicalensis* (Chinese skullcap)
>
> *Alchornea cordifolia*
>
> *Polygonum cuspidatum* (Japanese knotweed)[4]

Finally, we cannot ignore *Bartonella*. It may be more common than Lyme disease, and *Bartonella* can cause hundreds of medical and psychiatric problems. *Bartonella* is carried by many types of insects—not merely ticks. Herbs that kill *Bartonella* bacteria include:

> *Cryptolepis sanguinolenta*
>
> *Juglans nigra* (Black walnut)
>
> *Polygonum cuspidatum* (Japanese knotweed)

Herbs that Kill All Three—Lyme, Babesia, and Bartonella

Y. Zhang found that at least four herbs kill Lyme, *Babesia*, and *Bartonella*.

(*Cryptolepis sanguinolenta*) - Return Healthy Brand

Black walnut (*Juglans nigra*) - Horbaach Brand

Japanese knotweed (*Polygonum cuspidatum*) - Purity Labs Trans-resveratrol

Chinese skullcap (*Scutellaria baicalensis*) - Horbaach Brand

The Good News

A number of natural treatments appear to defeat Lyme, *Babesia,* and *Bartonella,* if test-tube studies are trustworthy. It would not surprise me if a million people have tried each of these herbs throughout the world over at least hundreds of years.

Finally, you should know that those who prescribe herbs like to use more than one herb. This benefit is like using 1 plus 1 plus 1 to equal 10.

Now let us look at these winning herbs before you blindly use them.

Cryptolepis sanguinolenta

Cryptolepis is amazing. It is an antibiotic, antiviral, antifungal, and antiparasitic treatment.[5] It will even bake cookies for you.

It can, however, lower fertility in both genders. It should not be used with patients trying to get pregnant.[6] This is why some healers only use it for short periods of time. My opinion is that it is wise to consult a herbal medicine expert if you are trying to get pregnant or are pregnant. This may apply to both men and women.

In 2021, Dr. Y. Zhang did test-tube studies that amazingly showed that only a weak, 1% potency of *Cryptolepis sanguinolenta* extract caused complete eradication of Lyme.[3] Other herbs and two traditional antibiotics were not this powerful against Lyme, because after three weeks, the Lyme bacteria were still visible.[2]

Finally, *Cryptolepis* has an unpleasant taste. So, my patients prefer it with glycerin as a liquid or as a capsule. Just be sure to check the date on the capsules since you want fresh ones.

Japanese Knotweed
(*Polygonum cuspidatum*)

Japanese knotweed is strong enough to treat Lyme in the brain and heart. It may reduce "die-off" or Herx reactions. A "Herx" (Herxheimer reaction) is discomfort after an effective herb kills an infection and the resulting debris creates strong body inflammation and a strong immune response that feels miserable. Surprisingly, Japanese knotweed blocks some of the excess inflammation from infections. It stops some of the inflammatory chemicals called "cytokines." Knotweed is the only herb that blocks MMP-1 and MMP-3.[7]

Japanese knotweed is protective of brain nerves. It also contains resveratrol, specifically, *trans*-resveratrol which is the most useful part for eliminating your infections. Resveratrol is pure **standardized** Japanese knotweed. Buhner suggests not using resveratrol from grapes.

Top herbalist Stephen Buhner suggests using this herb to treat both Lyme and *Bartonella*. In his *Bartonella* textbook, he also says Japanese knotweed protects the fragile lining of your blood vessels which *Bartonella* clearly infects.[8] Zhang has shown that it treats growing and persister states of Lyme and *Bartonella*.[9] This is a big deal, but only if you comprehend the power of persister cells. It has been said that after a nuclear bomb only cockroaches would survive. After antibiotics wipe out much Lyme and *Bartonella* bacteria, it is not all gone. The Lyme and *Bartonella* persisters remain. And Japanese knotweed helps defeat them. This is exciting since some people relapse because of hardy persisters.[10, 11]

A typical dose for an adult is 200 mg twice a day for three days and increase every two days for a top dose of 800 mg twice or three times a day (Modified from Dr. Bill Rawls).[15] Stephen Buhner suggests a tincture for three different infections of 1 tsp. 3 to 6 times a day. In his *Bartonella* book he suggests one capsule 3 times a day (Green Dragon Botanicals).[10]

Andrographis
(*Andrographis paniculata*)

Andrographis treats many viruses, such as the flu, COVID 19, and Hepatitis B and C. It also kills harsh bacteria like E. coli. Surprisingly, it also kills roundworms and tapeworms. H. Zhang reports that it has **anti-tumor, anti-bacterial, anti-inflammation, anti-virus, anti-fibrosis, anti-obesity** activity and according to Okhuarobo, it also kills malaria and protozoa—these are single celled parasites like *Babesia*.[12, 13]

Okhuarobo reviewed all major research on safety and concluded: the results of numerous toxicity evaluations of extracts and metabolites isolated from this plant did not show any significant acute toxicity in experimental animals.[13]

In Buhner's book Healing Lyme, he reports andrographolide is effective against Lyme in 60% of those ill with this infection.[14]

Rawls suggests using *Andrographis* in adults at 200 to 800 mg as an extract standardized to 10-30% *Andrographis*.[15] Start with one dose each day for three days and then take it twice a day. Tang reports a daily dose of 600 to 1,800 mg of the extract to treat ulcerative colitis in a human study.[16] Sometimes an ingredient is listed as "10% Andrographolides." Andrographolides are the effective herbal chemical in this herb. Buhner suggests 600 mg capsules 3 times a day for a week and suggests increasing to 1200 mg 3 times a day if tolerated. It tends to have more side effects than other natural treatments.[14]

Finally, if you are having inflammation labs done at Radiance labs (LH 14) and National Jewish Health (TH1/TH2 Panel A **only)**, your doctor may be able to track the inflammation chemicals making you miserable. The National Jewish Health website does not show this panel clearly—your doctor will need to set up an account. In the laboratory, Sandborn found *Andrographis* lowers TNF-α, IL-1β and NF-κB. The ability to target cytokines or inflammation precisely is exciting.[17]

Since it tastes so bitter, some practitioners suggest putting it in capsules.

In a Thailand study, the only side effects were increased immune system cells, a lower alkaline phosphatase, a rise in urine pH, and a brief decrease in blood pressure.[18] No person experienced serious side effects.

Houttuynia cordata

About eighteen years ago, I met and became friends with the leading Chinese herbalist in America—Dr. QingCai Zhang. After our initial meeting in Philadelphia, QingCai flew to Naples, Florida to discuss the high purity of his herbs and his exhaustive quality testing. And then he listened to my self-funded research on the effectiveness of two of his herbs—including HH or *Houttuynia cordata*. Simply, I found that three HH per day was not strong enough to kill most *Bartonella*. So, Dr. Zhang doubled the potency and called it HH2. His press release said, "Dr. James Schaller has done clinical observations and found that with higher dosage, the therapeutic efficacy improves. He suggested [we] produce a double strength version…Now the double strength HH2 Capsule [is available.]"

Over the last fifteen years my research suggested this herb is good at hindering *Bartonella* and lowering the number of *Bartonella* bacteria. But I do not believe it is typically curative at any dose, since at very high doses for a year you can still see *Bartonella* on a blood smear.

Currently, you can purchase this from Dr. Zhang's son, Dr. Yale Zhang at the Zhang Clinic NYC. It is now called "HH-M."

Zhang Clinic
(914) 259-0346

Or purchase online
DrRons.com

One possible option is to use the essential oil of *Houttuynia* after it is tested aggressively for purity and safety. Not all brands are pure. It is already in use for many antiviral and antibiotic purposes, according to Pang.[19]

Finally, with all the excellent biological uses of *Houttuynia*, please note it also lowers inflammation chemicals which likely contribute to your illness and discomfort. If your doctor is using Radiance Labs and National Jewish Health to measure inflammatory cytokines, look for the *Houttuynia* herb or its essential oil to reduce TNF-α, IL-1β, IL-6 and IL-8.[20] If you use routine national labs to measure special inflammation chemicals, cytokines, interferons, and interleukins, you will only get negatives over and over again—even if you are very ill.

Cat's Claw (Samento or *Uncaria tomentosa*)

Cat's Claw has been used for thousands of years by the people of the Amazon. The inner root or vine bark is the source of this herb.

It has strong anti-inflammatory benefits and calms excess immune reactivity.[21] It is used for high blood pressure, asthma, cancer, diabetes, arthritis, and neurodegenerative diseases. More than 200 compounds have been isolated from *Uncaria*.

This herb is used by natural healers for Lyme disease. But only limited research supports this use. Even PubMed, with tens of millions of medical studies, showed only one looking at Lyme and *Uncaria* together, authored by Feng.[2] Zhang and Feng showed Cat's Claw is one of the top herbs in the treatment of Lyme disease.[21]

Finally, do not use if you are pregnant, and be aware some people have nausea, belly spasms, and diarrhea.

Adult dosing is 400 to 800 mg of inner bark standardized to 3% alkaloids or 10:1 concentration of the inner bark (Rawls).[15] Buhner suggests a 1:5 concentration in 60% alcohol at about 50 drops taken 1-3 doses a day. It should be taken with food, according to Rawls, because stomach acid makes it work.[22]

Otoba parvifolia (Banderol)

At a recent conference on Lyme, *Babesia*, and *Bartonella*, a number of doctors reported using Banderol with success. Years ago, I did self-funded research on this herb. I was unable to come to a conclusion. And on PubMed, little existed on this extract. However, the combination of *Otaba parvifolia* (Banderol) with *Uncaria tomentosa* (Cat's Claw) was evaluated for its ability to kill Lyme in a lab. Extracts from these two plants were tested for their effectiveness on active and dormant forms of *Borrelia burgdorferi* (a species of Lyme) demonstrating significant effects on all its forms, especially when used in **combination**.[23]

Artemisia, Artesunate and Artemisinin

If you really want to learn about this family of herbs, please see my free book offered on personalconsult.com. It is the #1 book on Amazon.com on this topic.[24]

One concern I have is that some doctors prescribe the plain, unchanged herb *Artemisia* to kill *Babesia*. I reported in 2006 that the plain *Artemisia* herb is too weak to kill *Babesia*.[24] Elfawal found that both *Artemisia annua* and Artemisinin did not kill *Babesia*.[25]

Artemisia annua has been used for millennia to treat parasites and fever-related ailments caused by various infections.[25] Although effective against many infectious agents, the plant is not a miracle cure and there are infections where it has proved ineffective or of limited value. It is important to report those failures. For example, *Artemisia annua*, artesunate, and artemisinin were ineffective in reducing or eliminating *Babesia* in infected mice. Therefore, if you use potent semisynthetic artesunate, try to take a high dose and never believe one treatment will kill your *Babesia*.

Also, it should be mentioned that *Artemisia annua* has an essential oil.[26] These can be very strong treatments. My only concern is it has a significant amount of camphor, which is in many cold and flu medications that are available without a prescription. Camphor is in Vicks inhaler, Tiger balm, some Emu oils, and Vicks VapoRub.

Currently I would start with two capsules of artemisinin 100 mg to 200 mg twice a day for five days to see if you are sensitive to this mild treatment. For example, many people with Lyme, *Babesia,* and *Bartonella* can develop reactive mast cells which carry about 1000 chemicals which can make you feel poorly. If you do react, use weak *Artemisia* herb with no alteration so it does not make a large amount of *Babesia* die-off debris that fires up the immune system to make inflammation chemicals. However, if you tolerate artemisinin at 100 mg to 200 mg, double the dose after five days to 200 mg to 400 mg per day.

Then move to the much more powerful artesunate. Purchase this from www.DrRons.com. They offer a fairly strong form that was made twice as strong based on my research (Q. Zhang). Now it is called "Arte-M." Also, some doctors like to administer artesunate into your muscle or by IV. One possible dose is 120 mg.

My friend Henri Lindner, an exceptional *Babesia* scholar, and I have independently settled on artesunate as one very useful way to kill *Babesia*. And it seems this was accepted many years ago—artesunate is superior to artemisinin according to Jansen.[28] (However, we both strongly believe that using a single herb or synthetic treatment will not cure you of *Babesia*). I suggested this in my six *Babesia* books in 2006, but Lindner extended this hunch with great clinical creativity and has proved it clinically.

The essential oil of *Artemisia annua,* consisting of camphor (44%), germacrene D (16%), was screened for its antimicrobial activity. The essential oil remarkably inhibited the growth of tested gram-positive bacteria.[27] Camphor should be used carefully and not regularly, because it is a neurotoxin.

IV or Muscle-Injected Artesunate

Artesunate for injection is the treatment for severe malaria in adult and child patients.[29]

Artesunate for injection, 110 mg or 120 mg is intended for intravenous administration. In 2022 the CDC and FDA approved IV use of artesunate for cases of severe malaria and strongly recommended it be stocked in ERs and other locations with possible malaria patients.[30]

Why am I discussing a malaria drug that might work very fast? My good friend, Valerie Viale Fuller, founder of Band Aid Lyme, LLC, repeatedly almost died from *Babesia* many times. No one thought to give her IV artesunate. In my opinion, *Babesia* is much harder to kill than malaria.

Currently, a pharmaceutical company is being aggressive in trying to get IV artesunate distributed widely. Here are their home page comments:

> No FDA-approved injectable malaria medication has been available in the US since IV quinidine was discontinued in early 2019. Artesunate for injection fills this need.
>
> Healthcare professionals [having] difficulties obtaining products from our distributors should contact the Amivas Medical Affairs line below. This line is open 24/7/365:
>
> **AMIVAS MEDICAL AFFAIRS**
> **1-855-5AMIVAS**

Artesunate for injection, manufactured by Amivas, is approved by the FDA and is commercially available in the United States.

FDA-approved artesunate is available for purchase from major drug distributors.

The CDC mentions that "artesunate for injection can be given in infants, children, adults, and pregnant women.[31] IV artesunate can cause serious red blood cell problems which require transfusion. So, they suggest after giving artesunate IV, monitor patients starting at 7 days and up to 4 weeks after receiving intravenous artesunate is recommended." https://www.cdc.gov/malaria/new_info/2020/artesunate_approval.htm

Much of the world uses Artemisinin-based combination therapies (ACT) against *Babesia's* cousin, malaria. But what is ACT? It is the use of an *Artemisia* derivative combined with a different synthetic malaria killer.

The World Health Organization is strongly supporting using a herb and a synthetic drug together and these are called "artemisinin-based combination therapies" which are now being used in more than 50 countries where malaria is common. Therefore, we have massive experience using herbs with synthetic malaria drugs. **All *Babesia* treatments are malaria treatments**.

This is a possible lesson that I hope flows from this book. Using herbs and essential oils together with synthetic pharmacy medicine might often be useful in killing malaria, but also *Babesia*. The latter can be fatal or cause sweats, chills, headaches, air hunger or significant fatigue.

So let us look over Price's summary below, as he lists herb and drug combinations that are effective.[32]

The most common combinations to kill malaria are:

- artemether-lumefantrine (Coartem)

- artesunate-amodiaquine (Currently it is not available in USA or UK, but it can be acquired by Canadians under the Health Canada Special Access Program. This is associated with the Canadian malaria network. My good friend Ian, the top pharmacist at Kripps pharmacy in Canada, reported one would have to prove a need).

- artesunate-sulfadoxine-pyrimethamine (Fansidar).

- artesunate-mefloquine (mefloquine is Larium).

- dihydroartemisinin-piperaquine—Janson reports that dihydroartemisinic acid is **very unstable** and decomposes too easily. So, despite its potency, it has limitations.

The consensus from my discussions with *Babesia* literate physicians is that the herbal derivative artemether in the Coartem combination drug with lumefantrine is very well tolerated. The herbal part is artemether, which is synthetic. Many Lyme literate doctors prescribe eight tablets a day for three days—a bit aggressive. Personally, I have never had a patient have side effects on Coartem at any dose.

Garlic and Synthetic Garlic

Garlic oil helps eliminate *Babesia duncani*. Dr. Yumin Zhang found in lab experiments that routine CDC treatment with atovaquone (Mepron) and azithromycin (Zithromax) killed some *Babesia*, but with **relapse**.[33] This fact seems to be ignored by some *Babesia* researchers who seem to be unable to update this one treatment approach to killing *Babesia*. But adding garlic oil to azithromycin (Zithromax) killed the *Babesia* without any relapse. I have been using garlic, garlic oil, or semi-synthetic garlic for about twenty-nine years. The primary side effect is a strong body smell and possible mild stomach upset.

So how can you benefit from garlic oil?

It is best to start slowly with sensitive people using a simple garlic called "Allimed." Dr. L. Robert Mozayeni, the *Bartonella* expert, suggests this product. I agree. If that goes well at high dosing, move to garlic oil. You do not want to use an essential oil or semi-synthetic garlic yet. Use a plain garlic oil. Brands to consider are Puritans Pride or Nature's Way.

But please notice that many garlic supplements are "odorless." Avoid these products because the strong smell is a sign you are taking a brand that works.

This is a careful and gentle approach. Start with regular garlic or Allimed. Then move to a gentle oil. And then consider a semisynthetic powerful garlic medicine called "allicin" from the Zhang clinic in NYC. This is the best approach if you are sensitive to medications, have mast cell activation syndrome (MCAS), PANDAS or PANS.

Eventually, the goal is to have you take semisynthetic garlic from the Zhang Clinic. In 2006, I read QingCai Zhang's book on Chinese medicine to treat Lyme, *Babesia*, and *Bartonella*. And then I spent hours with him in Florida learning the extensive purity testing he used, but he also emphasized the potency of his special semi-synthetic garlic, which I believe saved the life of his son when given intravenously decades earlier in China.

Simply, order the allicin product from the Zhang Clinic in NYC. But please understand that while Q. Zhang's product is called "allicin," it is not simply regular garlic. To illustrate the potency, note that one small capsule will give you a profound garlic smell for 36 hours. Y. Zhang found that garlic essential oil had profound action against *Babesia*.[33]

Finally, Y. Zhang, at Johns Hopkins, routinely publishes pearls for the treatment of Lyme, *Babesia*, and *Bartonella*. In 2020, Y. Zhang and his team identified essential oils with high activity against *Babesia duncani*.[33] They screened 97 essential oils and identified **garlic oil as a top treatment to remove *Babesia*.**

Black Walnut
(*Juglans nigra*)

Black walnut was also shown to reduce *Borrelia burgdorferi* in test tubes by the Zhang team at Johns Hopkins.

Feng found a mere 1% extract of Black walnut had better activity against *B. burgdorferi* (a common species of Lyme disease bacteria) compared to the antibiotics doxycycline and cefuroxime in a lab study.[2]

Initially, I was not finding much on this herb regarding its antibiotic abilities—in many top naturopath textbooks, herbal textbooks and PubMed's 34 million articles. But, in addition to Feng's report that mentioned its strong effects against *Borrelia*, Black walnut is mentioned in The Naturopathic Herbalist in which naturopath Dr. Marisa Marciano reports benefits against bacteria, bacteria dispersed throughout the body, and yeast infections (and even treats parasitic worms).[34] It can be a laxative, so high dosing might cause loose stool.

Naphthoquinone juglone, one of the active components in Black walnut, is antifungal, a toxin, antimicrobial, and antiparasitic. The suggested tincture is 1:4, 25% with 5-10 drops three times a day with a maximum dose of 15 mL a week. She suggests doing two weeks on and two weeks off. Woodland Essence suggests a dosing of 10-30 drops, or 1/8 - 1/4 tsp 3 times per day in juice or water.[35]

Ho reported that Black walnut extract may lower inflammatory chemicals called cytokines; lowering the levels of certain cytokines might make you feel better.[36] While there was variation among varieties, as a trend Black walnut lowered inflammatory chemicals or cytokines. She concludes: "The results of this study demonstrated for the first time that Black walnut possesses compounds [to lower] six measured cytokines (TNF-α, IL-1β, IL-6, IL-8, IL-10, and MCP-1)."[36] This research used human cells stimulated by a very common bacterial chemical (LPS) which causes profound immune reactivity. Therefore, an effective dose of black walnut can cause aggressive killing of the infectious agents, but the inflammation may be less with this herb because the cultivated plants used for Ho's research lowered the cytokine "gasoline." Specifically, Black walnut reduced between one cytokine to as many as six of these inflammatory chemicals, depending on which subtype of plant was used for the extract.

Alchornea cordifolia

Alchornea cordifolia extracts showed good inhibitory effect against *Babesia duncani* according to Zhang.[3] It has antimicrobial and anti-inflammatory activity.[37, 38, 39, 40] *Alchornea cordifolia* has been used by traditional herbalists in several African countries for the treatment of malaria[41] [which is similar to *Babesia*]. Studies suggest significant antimalarial effects.[42, 43, 44]

The active constituents of *Alchornea cordifolia* extract are complex, including ellagic acid, and quercetin.[41] Ellagic acid has previously been shown in the lab to fight against malaria.[45,46] But it also might become a new herbal product to consider to kill *Babesia*.

Ellagic acid (EA) is found in various plant products and has antioxidant, antibacterial and effective antimalarial activity in the lab and the body without toxicity.[47] Ellagic acid can kill *Babesia*. If you wish to try this herbal extract, look at Pomegranate Extract 500 mg with whole fruit Ellagic Acid from Source Naturals.

Essential Oils Used Against Lyme, Babesia, and Bartonella

Among the 250 essential oils which are commercially available, about a dozen possess high antimicrobial activity.[50] Ma argues that the current treatment for *Bartonella* infections is not very effective due to antibiotic resistance and also persistence.[48] He tried 32 essential oils against *Bartonella*. The most effective *Bartonella* death happened with the essential oil of oregano, cinnamon bark, mountain savory (winter), cinnamon leaf, geranium, clove bud, allspice, geranium bourbon, ylang-ylang, citronella, elemi, and vetiver. **Carvacrol and cinnamaldehyde, the active ingredients of oil of oregano and cinnamon bark oil, respectively, were able to remove *Bartonella* totally even at low doses.**

Feng also reports some thoughts about essential oils.[49] He looked at 34 essential oils against *Borrelia burgdorferi* (Lyme). First, he quotes Wińska who found that not all essential oils had activity against the Lyme bacteria. But they did find five essential oils (oregano, cinnamon bark, clove bud, citronella, and wintergreen) which even at low doses killed the hard to remove persister cells of Lyme. Interestingly, some highly active essential oils were found to have excellent anti-biofilm ability—they dissolved the biofilm-like structures. I published similar positions in 2014 in my free textbook Combating Biofilms. I reported in 2014 that select essential oils—particularly oregano, cinnamon, and clove bud—destroy Lyme biofilms. Combinations of essential oils work best, and the stomach has to be protected if one goes to a high dose. Soothing Protective Herbs are marshmallow root, aloe vera in capsules, and slippery elm (Nature's Way is cost effective and useful). I have not seen one that is better than another. Consider using one stomach herb for a week and then switching to another.

Amazingly, **oils of oregano, cinnamon bark, and clove bud completely eradicated all viable Lyme bacteria without any regrowth**. *Citronella* and wintergreen were not as effective. Carvacrol in oregano oil had excellent activity against Lyme.

In 2020, Y. Zhang and his research team identified essential oils with high activity against *Babesia duncani*.[33] They screened 97 essential oils in the lab, and identified ten that were effective against *Babesia* and further narrowed their search for the two most effective compounds – **garlic oil and black pepper oil**. They also found that the routine recommended treatment for *Babesia* can have relapses. Specifically, **atovaquone liquid (Mepron) and azithromycin (Zithromax) at high dosing can allow the *Babesia* to return.** In contrast, the combination of garlic oil and azithromycin showed eradication of *Babesia* at low dosing.

Goc investigated 47 fats and oils, testing them against moving *Borrelia* (Lyme spirochetes) as well as the round-shaped persister cells that survive common antibiotics used in the treatment of Lyme disease.[51] These bacteria are protected by a strong protective slime or biofilm layer. Only bay leaf oil and Cassia oil, which have **eugenol and cinnamaldehyde**, destroyed different stages of Lyme disease and also its protective biofilm. I made a similar report in my 2014 textbook Combating Biofilms.[52]

One helpful study investigated volatile oils including three essential oils: oregano oil, cinnamon oil, and clove oil. All three were even more powerful than daptomycin, an antibiotic shown to kill *Borrelia's* persisters. These Lyme cells are usually alive and "persisting" after full antibiotic treatment. And then slowly patients feel the Lyme disease returning.

A practical issue in using essential oils is what brand to use and what is the daily dose taken with food? After twenty-five years of use, I doubt a very low dose will do much. For example, I have seen good results with the application of clovanol to infected gums applied most evenings. But I do not believe this dose on the gums enters your blood stream, and kills pathogens, such as *Borrelia, Babesia,* and *Bartonella*, in your joints, intestines, or brain.

Cinnamol is a compound I have used since 1998 because it defeats the protective biofilms routinely seen with infections—biofilms make common antibiotics fail.[53] A biofilm may make killing the bacteria twenty times harder to remove. Moreover, this substance suppresses the *Candida* species and its biofilm. When I was learning the basics long ago—none of this information was clear.

But perhaps you are wondering exactly how the top essential oils are taken? Are they put into a nebulizer to spread mist throughout the nasal cavity? No. There are a number of high quality essential oil companies. But all my self-funded research has been with the products made by North American Herb and Spice. Typically, I have patients buy three products: oreganol gel balls, clovanol liquid and cinnamol liquid. I typically have patients slowly add two oreganol gell balls three times a day to meals and increase if tolerated.

The clovanol and cinnamon liquids are placed inside the capsules with **stomach-protective herb powder**. My patients buy inexpensive Nature's Way Marshmallow Root, Aloe Vera capsules, or Slippery Elm. Take one of these three protective stomach herbs and open the capsule. So, for example, take a Marshmallow Root capsule, pull it apart, and discard half the powder. Next, drop in the essential oil into the open capsule space. Close up the capsule. The hope is that the stomach will be fine. I typically start with one drop three times a day with reactive, sensitive people, those with mast cell syndrome, PANDAS or PANS. If this starting oil dose does not bother your stomach, I increase it by a drop every two days. With enough stomach protective herbs, most patients are able to reach ten drops, always taken with your three daily meals. I rotate my three favorite essential oils mentioned above, so all are used in three days.

Chinese skullcap (*Scutellaria baicalensis* or *Calvaria*)

One principle promoted by my natural medicine doctor friends is the benefit of combining herbs. In Chinese skullcap, we have a herb that **improves the absorption of other herbs. This is an amazing feature.**

It is also a good antiviral. And ticks carry a number of viruses like Epstein-Barr, Parvo, Mycoplasma pneumoniae, HHV6 (a herpes virus), Coxsackie, and SARS-CoV-2, which causes COVID-19.

It is good for calming allergies, autoimmunity, and is protective of nerves. Since Lyme disease, *Babesia,* and *Bartonella* can cause all three problems, it is a nice option.

But this herb is also a top killer of three forms of Lyme disease, such as the active spiral bacteria, round persister forms, and biofilm-protected bacteria hiding behind a protective slime.[54]

Cistus incanus (or *Cistus creticus*)

Some people believe *Cistus creticus* and *Cistus incanus* are the same herb. Clinical studies show the volatile oil extract of *Cistus creticus* to have antibiotic and **anti-borrelial effects in the lab.**[2] Additional lab studies have shown *Cistus creticus* to have broad and effective antimicrobial effects against several bacteria. *Cistus creticus* also defeated a *Strep* biofilm.

Cistus incanus plant extracts have been used for centuries in traditional medicine without reports of side effects or allergic reactions. In a randomized placebo-controlled study of 160 patients, 220 mg per day *Cistus incanus* was well tolerated with less adverse effects than in the placebo group.

Teasel

Dipsacus sylvestris is known as wild teasel or fuller's teasel. Its extracts have been studied against Lyme disease in the lab by Liebold. [55, 59] Teasel prevented all growth of the *Borrelia* spirochetes.

Wild teasel has been examined as a Lyme treatment.[56] Previously, all the anti-*Borrelia* research focused on the root, which is not effective against Lyme. However, the leaves demonstrate useful antimicrobial effects.[61]

Lowering "Herx" Reactions with Herbs

There are many articles promoting nutrition, saunas, lymph massage, hyperbaric treatment, binders, and dozens of other options to lower your discomfort caused by the infection die-off debris resulting from strong and effective herbs and essential oils. I will only discuss herbal Herx options.

In past discussions with Dr. QingCai Zhang, the leading USA Chinese Medicine expert, he believed his Puerarin-M herb could lower the discomfort of inflammatory debris from pathogen die-off resulting from effective treatment of infections.

I would try one Puerarin twice a day for three days and then one three times a day. It does not always work, but it is worth a try.

Purchase at:

Zhang Clinic
(914) 259-0346

Online availability
DrRons.com

Zhou reported the beneficial effects of Puerarin are due to dilation of blood vessels, heart protection, reduced inflammation, brain protection, calming free radicals, and lowering pain.[57] Therefore, this has potential to lower Herx pain. Try it for five weeks.

Chlorella

Years ago, I was hired to research a fascinating form of **pulverized** *Chlorella* as a toxin binder—particularly of heavy metals. *Chlorella* is a form of green algae, packed with many vitamins, minerals, and protein. It has also been proposed by Hirooka as a binder of **chemicals** that try to harm the body by resembling estrogen (called xenoestrogen where "xeno" means foreign).[58] These foreign estrogens may promote cancer. Some believe that chlorella may bind a wide variety of inflammatory chemicals, but that is for another book. In my research, I found that one product called NDF Organic from Bioray.com removed metals in hours, not days. Try a full dropper the instant you wake up before eating or drinking. You do not want it merely removing toxins in your food. You may lose some heavy metals and chemical xeno-estrogens that cause cancer.[58] And it might bind inflammatory chemicals and toxins from die-off debris.

Dandelion Root

Dandelion root is believed to promote the liver's role to help remove inflammatory chemicals which cause discomfort. Gonzalez-Castejon reported that the evidence suggests that dandelion root's many plant chemicals have antioxidant and anti-inflammatory activities in many areas of the body.[59]

Modified Citrus Pectin

Try to start with 3, two times a day at least 90 minutes away from food or herbs. Consider using Pectasol brand.

Modified citrus pectin lowers or removes heavy metals and possibly infection die-off debris. There are extensive publications about its use as a supplement important in breast, prostate, and melanoma cancer treatment. It inhibits Galectin-3 which may promote cancer relapse and tumor progression. (Source: DrEliaz.com)

Optifiber Lean

Nathan, quoting J. Callahan, suggests that Optifiber Lean may be a very strong binder.[60] I have no opinion. I do wonder if some binders, like cholestyramine, lower fat-soluble vitamins as they bind fatty chemicals. I am still studying this issue, but doubt it is a routine problem.

Japanese Knotweed

Japanese knotweed has a calming effect on the infected body. Japanese knotweed blocks some of the excess inflammation from infections. It stops some of the inflammatory chemicals called "cytokines." For example, knotweed is the only herb that lowers MMP-1 and MMP-3 in a mouse study.[7] Knotweed is highly active impacting MMP-9, lowering IL-6 and TNF-α, and possibly altering COX-2. Resveratrol from knotweed has a protective effect against sun damage in mice, and some think this might occur in human cells.

Cannabis Derivatives

CBD, CBG, and THC from cannabis require a look at how cannabis impacts Herx reactions.[61] Tumor necrosis factor alpha (TNF-a), interleukin (IL)-1β, IL-6, and interferon gamma were the most commonly studied pro-inflammatory chemicals and their levels were consistently reduced after treatment with CBD, CBG, or a CBD+THC combination, but not with THC alone. In 22 studies, in which CBD, CBG, or CBD in combination with THC were administered, at least one inflammatory chemical was reduced. And, in 24 studies, there were some improvements in disease or disability. THC alone did not reduce pro-inflammatory cytokine levels…but resulted in improvements in neuropathic pain in one study.[61]

CBD, CBG, and a CBD+THC combination exert a predominantly anti-inflammatory effect in bodies (not merely in laboratories).[61]

Quercetin

Quercetin is an example of an anti-inflammatory plant pigment that lowers cytokines, such as interleukin-1 beta (IL-1β), tumor necrosis factor-alpha (TNF-α), interleukin-6 (IL-6), and interleukin-8 (IL-8).[62] These are best evaluated by Radiance Labs 14 cytokine inflammation panel and/or National Jewish Health laboratory advanced inflammation chemicals TH1/TH2 Panel A. Physicians can only access the latter by calling them, since this precise panel does not exist on their website. Your sample has to be shipped on ice and the panel costs approximately $280.00. Using other routine, national laboratories to measure levels of advanced cytokines, interleukins and interferons, is a complete waste of time.

ENDNOTES

1. Gadila S, Embers ME. Antibiotic Susceptibility of *Bartonella* Grown in Different Culture Conditions. Pathogens. 2021 Jun 8;10(6):718. doi: 10.3390/pathogens10060718. PMID: 34201011 PMCID: PMC8229624.

2. Feng J, Leone J, Schweig S, and Zhang Y. Evaluation of Natural and Botanical Medicines for Activity Against Growing and Non-growing Forms of *B. burgdorferi*. Front. Med., 21 February 2020 Sec. Infectious Diseases – Surveillance, Prevention and Treatment https://doi.org/10.3389/fmed.2020.00006

3. Zhang Y, Alvarez-Manzo H, Leone J, Schweig S and Zhang Y. (2021)Botanical Medicines *Cryptolepis sanguinolenta, Artemisia annua, Scutellaria baicalensis, Polygonumcuspidatum*, and *Alchornea cordifolia* Demonstrate Inhibitory Activity Against *Babesia duncani*. Front. Cell. Infect. Microbiol. 11:624745. doi: 10.3389/fcimb.2021.624745

4. Ma, Xiao; Leone, Jacob; Schweig, Sunjya; Zhang, Ying. Botanical Medicines With Activity Against Stationary Phase Bartonella henselae. Infectious Microbes & Diseases 3(3):p 158-167, September 2021. doi: 10.1097/IM9.0000000000000069

5. *Cryptolepis (Cryptolepis sanguinolenta)* — Herbal Monograph (thesunlightexperiment.com), Accessed November 3, 2022.

6. Ajayi AF, Akhigbe RE. Antifertility activity of *Cryptolepis sanguinolenta* leaf ethanolic extract in male rats. J Hum Reprod Sci. 2012 Jan;5(1):43-7.

7. Cui B, Wang Y, Jin J, Yang Z, Guo R, Li X, Yang L, Li Z. Resveratrol Treats UVB-Induced Photoaging by Anti-MMP Expression, through Anti-Inflammatory, Antioxidant, and Antiapoptotic Properties, and Treats Photoaging by Upregulating VEGF-B Expression. Oxid Med Cell Longev. 2022 Jan 4;2022:6037303. doi: 10.1155/2022/6037303. PMID: 35028009; PMCID: PMC8752231.

8. Buhner, S. Healing Lyme Disease Coinfections: Complementary and Holistic Treatments for *Bartonella* and *Mycoplasma*. May 5, 2013, Healing Arts Press, Rochester VT.

9. Zhang H, Li C, Kwok ST, Zhang QW, Chan SW. A Review of the Pharmacological Effects of the Dried

Root of *Polygonum cuspidatum* (Hu Zhang) and Its Constituents. Evid Based Complement Alternat Med. 2013;2013:208349. doi: 10.1155/2013/208349. Epub 2013 Sep 30. PMID: 24194779; PMCID: PMC3806114. (Hidawi)

10. Buhner, S. Herbal Antibiotics, 2nd Edition: Natural Alternatives for Treating Drug-resistant Bacteria. Jul 17, 2012 Storey Publishing, North Adams MA. pp. 61, 70, 72.

11. Buhner, S. Natural Treatments for Lyme Coinfections: *Anaplasma*, *Babesia*, and *Ehrlichia*. Feb 22, 2015. Healing Arts Press, Rochester VT. pp. 219—224.

12. Zhang H, Li S, Si Y, Xu H. Andrographolide and its derivatives: Current achievements and future perspectives. Eur J Med Chem. 2021 Nov 15;224:113710. doi: 10.1016/j.ejmech.2021.113710. Epub 2021 Jul 20. PMID: 34315039.

13. Okhuarobo A, Faludun JE, Erharuyi O, Imieje V, Falodun A, Langer P. Harnessing the medicinal properties of *Andrographis paniculata* for diseases and beyond: a review of its phytochemistry and pharmacology. Asian Pac J Trop Dis. 2014 Jun; 4(3): 213–222. doi: 10.1016/S2222-1808(14)60509-0

14. Buhner, S and Nathan N. Healing Lyme: Natural Healing of Lyme Borreliosis and the Coinfections

Chlamydia and Spotted Fever Rickettsiosis, 2nd Edition. Dec 7, 2015. Raven Press. pp. 204, 215.

15. Rawls, B. The Cellular Wellness Solution: Tap Into Your Full Health Potential with the Science-Backed Power of Herbs. June 18, 2022, First Do No Harm Publishing, Raleigh NC.

16. Tang T, Targan SR, Li ZS, Xu C, Byers VS, Sandborn WJ. Randomised clinical trial: herbal extract HMPL-004 in active ulcerative colitis - a double-blind comparison with sustained release mesalazine. Aliment Pharmacol Ther. 2011 Jan;33(2):194-202. doi: 10.1111/j.1365-2036.2010.04515.x. Epub 2010 Nov 30. PMID: 21114791.

17. Sandborn WJ, Targan SR, Byers VS, Rutty DA, Mu H, Zhang X, Tang T. *Andrographis paniculata* extract (HMPL-004) for active ulcerative colitis. Am J Gastroenterol. 2013 Jan;108(1):90-8. doi: 10.1038/ajg.2012.340. Epub 2012 Oct 9. PMID: 23044768; PMCID: PMC3538174.

18. Suriyo T, Pholphana N, Ungtrakul T, Rangkadilok N, Panomvana D, Thiantanawat A, Pongpun W, Satayavivad J. Clinical Parameters following Multiple Oral Dose Administration of a Standardized *Andrographis paniculata* Capsule in Healthy Thai Subjects. Planta Med. 2017 Jun;83(9):778-789.

doi: 10.1055/s-0043-104382. Epub 2017 Mar 1. PMID: 28249303.

19. Pang J, Dong W, Li Y, Xia X, Liu Z, Hao H, Jiang L, Liu Y. Purification of *Houttuynia cordata Thunb.* Essential Oil Using Macroporous Resin Followed by Microemulsion Encapsulation to Improve Its Safety and Antiviral Activity. Molecules. 2017 Feb 15;22(2):293. doi: 10.3390/molecules22020293. PMID: 28212296; PMCID: PMC6155675.

20. Laldinsangi C. The therapeutic potential of *Houttuynia cordata*: A current review. Heliyon. 2022 Aug 24;8(8):e10386. doi: 10.1016/j.heliyon.2022. e10386. PMID: 36061012; PMCID: PMC9433674.

21. Zhang Q, Zhao JJ, Xu J, Feng F, Qu W. Medicinal uses, phytochemistry and pharmacology of the genus *Uncaria*. J Ethnopharmacol. 2015 Sep 15;173:48-80. doi: 10.1016/j.jep.2015.06.011. Epub 2015 Jun 17. PMID: 26091967.

22. Buhner, S. Herbal Antibiotics, 2nd Edition: Natural Alternatives for Treating Drug-resistant Bacteria. Jul 17, 2012 Storey Publishing, North Adams MA. p. 379.

23. Goc A, Rath M. The anti-borreliae efficacy of phytochemicals and micronutrients: an update. Ther Adv Infect Dis. 2016 Jun;3(3-4):75-82. doi: 10.1177/

2049936116655502. Epub 2016 Jul 4. PMID: 27536352; PMCID: PMC4971593.

24. Schaller, J. Artemisinin, Artesunate, Artemisinic Acid and Other Derivatives of Artemisia Used for Malaria, Babesia and Cancer. October 13, 2006, Hope Academic Press, Tampa FL.

25. Elfawal MA, Gray O, Dickson-Burke C, Weathers PJ, Rich SM. *Artemisia* annua and artemisinins are ineffective against human *Babesia microti* and six *Candida* sp. Longhua Chin Med. 2021 Jun;4:12. doi: 10.21037/lcm-21-2. PMID: 34316676; PMCID: PMC8312716.

26. Juteau F, Masotti V, Bessière JM, Dherbomez M, Viano J. Antibacterial and antioxidant activities of *Artemisia annua* essential oil. Fitoterapia. 2002 Oct;73(6):532-5. doi: 10.1016/s0367-326x(02)00175-2. PMID: 12385883.

27. Bilia AR, Santomauro F, Sacco C, Bergonzi MC, Donato R. Essential Oil of *Artemisia annua* L.: An Extraordinary Component with Numerous Antimicrobial Properties. Evid Based Complement Alternat Med. 2014;2014:159819. doi: 10.1155/2014/159819. Epub 2014 Apr 1. PMID: 24799936; PMCID: PMC3995097.

28 Jansen FH. The pharmaceutical death-ride of dihydroartemisinin. Malar J. 2010 Jul 22;9:212. doi: 10.1186/1475-2875-9-212. PMID: 20649950; PMCID: PMC2916014.

29. https://www.rxlist.com/artesunate-drug.htm. Accessed November 3, 2022.

30. https://www.cdc.gov/malaria/diagnosis_treatment/discontinuation_artesunate.html.

31. https://www.cdc.gov/malaria/new_info/2020/artesunate_approval.htm. Accessed November 3, 2022.

32. Price RN, Douglas NM. Artemisinin combination therapy for malaria: beyond good efficacy. Clin Infect Dis. 2009 Dec 1;49(11):1638-40. doi: 10.1086/647947. PMID: 19877970; PMCID: PMC4627500.

33. Zhang Y, Bai C, Shi W, Alvarez-Manzo H, Zhang Y. Identification of Essential Oils Including Garlic Oil and Black Pepper Oil with High Activity against *Babesia duncani*. Pathogens. 2020 Jun 12;9(6):466. doi: 10.3390/pathogens9060466. PMID: 32545549; PMCID: PMC7350376.

34. https://thenaturopathicherbalist.com/herbs/i-l/juglans-nigra-black-walnut/ Marisa Marciano. Accessed November 3, 2022.

35. https://woodlandessence.com/products/black-walnut-liquid-extract. Accessed November 3, 2022.

36. Ho KV, Schreiber KL, Vu DC, Rottinghaus SM, Jackson DE, Brown CR, Lei Z, Sumner LW, Coggeshall MV, Lin CH. Black Walnut (*Juglans nigra*) Extracts Inhibit Proinflammatory Cytokine Production From Lipopolysaccharide-Stimulated Human Promonocytic Cell Line U-937. Front Pharmacol. 2019 Sep 19; 10:1059. doi: 10.3389/fphar.2019.01059. PMID: 31607915; PMCID: PMC6761373.

37. Ebi, G. C. (2001). Antimicrobial activities of *Alchornea cordifolia*. Fitoterapia 72, 69–72. doi: 10.1016/S0367-326X(00)00254-9

38. Manga, H. M., Brkic, D., Marie, D. E., and Quetin-Leclercq, J. (2004). In vivo antiinflammatory activity of *Alchornea cordifolia* (Schumach. Thonn.) Mull. Arg. (Euphorbiaceae). J. Ethnopharmacol. 92, 209–214. doi: 10.1016/ j.jep.2004.02.019

39. Shan, B., Cai, Y. Z., Brooks, J. D., and Corke, H. (2008). Antibacterial properties of *Polygonum cuspidatum* roots and their major bioactive constituents. Food Chem. 109, 530–537. doi: 10.1016/j.foodchem.2007.12.064

40. Ghanim, H., Sia, C. L., Abuaysheh, S., Korzeniewski, K., Patnaik, P., Marumganti, A., et al. (2010). An

antiinflammatory and reactive oxygen species suppressive effects of an extract of *Polygonum cuspidatum* containing resveratrol. J. Clin. Endocrinol. Metab. 95, E1–E8. doi: 10.1210/mend.24.7.9998

41. Boniface, P. K., Ferreira, S. B., and Kaiser, C. R. (2016). Recent trends in phytochemistry, ethnobotany and pharmacological significance of *Alchornea cordifolia* (Schumach. & Thonn.) Muell. Arg. J. Ethnopharmacol. 191, 216–244. doi: 10.1016/j.jep.2016.06.021

42. Mustofa, A., Benoit-Vical, F., Pelissier, Y., Kone-Bamba, D., and Mallie, M. (2000). Antiplasmodial activity of plant extracts used-in west African traditional medicine. J. Ethnopharmacol. 73, 145–151. doi: 10.1016/S0378-8741(00) 00296-8

43. Mesia, G. K., Tona, G. L., Nanga, T. H., Cimanga, R. K., Apers, S., Cos, P., et al. (2008). Antiprotozoal and cytotoxic screening of 45 plant extracts from Democratic Republic of Congo. J. Ethnopharmacol. 115, 409–415. doi: 10.1016/j.jep.2007.10.028

44. Ayisi, N. K., Appiah-Opong, R., Gyan, B., Bugyei, K., and Ekuban, F. (2011). *Plasmodium falciparum*: Assessment of Selectivity of Action of Chloroquine, *Alchornea cordifolia, Ficus polita,* and Other Drugs by a Tetrazolium-Based Colorimetric Assay. Malar. Res. Treat 2011, 816250. doi: 10.4061/2011/816250

45. Lamikanra, A., Ogundaini, A. O., and Ogungbamila, F. O. (1990). Antibacterial Constituents of *Alchornea-Cordifolia* Leaves. Phytother. Res. 4, 198–200. doi: 10.1002/ptr.2650040508

46. Banzouzi, J. T., Prado, R., Menan, H., Valentin, A., Roumestan, C., Mallie, M., et al. (2002). In vitro antiplasmodial activity of extracts of *Alchornea cordifolia* and identification of an active constituent: ellagic acid. J. Ethnopharmacol. 81, 399– 401. doi: 10.1016/S0378-8741(02)00121-6

47. Beshbishy AM, Batiha GE, Yokoyama N, Igarashi I. Ellagic acid microspheres restrict the growth of *Babesia* and *Theileria* in vitro and *Babesia microti* in vivo. Parasit Vectors. 2019 May 28;12(1):269. doi: 10.1186/s13071-019-3520-x. PMID: 31138282; PMCID: PMC6537213.

48. Ma X, Shi W, Zhang Y. Essential Oils with High Activity against Stationary Phase *Bartonella henselae*. Antibiotics (Basel). 2019 Nov 30;8(4):246. doi: 10.3390/antibiotics8040246. PMID: 31801196; PMCID: PMC6963529.

49. Feng J, Zhang S, Shi W, Zubcevik N, Miklossy J, Zhang Y. Selective Essential Oils from Spice or Culinary Herbs Have High Activity against Stationary Phase and Biofilm *Borrelia burgdorferi*. Front Med

(Lausanne). 2017 Oct 11;4:169. doi: 10.3389/fmed.2017.00169. PMID: 29075628; PMCID: PMC5641543.

50. Wińska K, Mączka W, Łyczko J, Grabarczyk M, Czubaszek A, Szumny A. Essential Oils as Antimicrobial Agents-Myth or Real Alternative? Molecules. 2019 Jun 5;24(11):2130. doi: 10.3390/molecules24112130. PMID: 31195752; PMCID: PMC6612361.

51. Goc A, Niedzwiecki A, Rath M. Anti-borreliae efficacy of selected organic oils and fatty acids. BMC Complement Altern Med. 2019 Feb 4;19(1):40. doi: 10.1186/s12906-019-2450-7. PMID: 30717726; PMCID: PMC6360722.

52. Schaller J, Mountjoy K. Combating Biofilms. April 11, 2014. International Infectious Disease Press. Naples FL.

53. Didehdar M, Chegini Z, Tabaeian SP, Razavi S, Shariati A. *Cinnamomum:* The New Therapeutic Agents for Inhibition of Bacterial and Fungal Biofilm-Associated Infection. Front Cell Infect Microbiol. 2022 Jul 8;12:930624. doi: 10.3389/fcimb.2022.930624. PMID: 35899044; PMCID: PMC9309250.

54. Goc A, Niedzwiecki A, Rath M. In vitro evaluation of antibacterial activity of phytochemicals and micronutrients against *Borrelia burgdorferi* and *Borrelia garinii*. J Appl Microbiol. 2015 Dec; 119(6):1561-72. doi: 10.1111/jam.12970. PMID: 26457476; PMCID: PMC4738477.

55. Liebold T, Straubinger RK, Rauwald HW. Growth inhibiting activity of lipophilic extracts from Dipsacus sylvestris Huds. roots against Borrelia burgdorferi s. s. in vitro. Pharmazie. 2011 Aug;66(8):628-30. PMID: 21901989.

56. Saar-Reismaa P, Bragina O, Kuhtinskaja M, Reile I, Laanet PR, Kulp M, Vaher M. Extraction and Fractionation of Bioactives from *Dipsacus fullonum* L. Leaves and Evaluation of Their Anti-*Borrelia* Activity. Pharmaceuticals (Basel). 2022 Jan 12;15(1):87. doi: 10.3390/ph15010087. PMID: 35056144; PMCID: PMC8779505.

57. Zhou YX, Zhang H, Peng C. Puerarin: a review of pharmacological effects. Phytother Res. 2014 Jul;28(7):961-75. doi: 10.1002/ptr.5083. Epub 2013 Dec 13. PMID: 24339367.

58. Hirooka T, Nagase H, Uchida K, Hiroshige Y, Ehara Y, Nishikawa J, Nishihara T, Miyamoto K, Hirata Z. Biodegradation of bisphenol A and

disappearance of its estrogenic activity by the green alga *Chlorella fusca* var. vacuolata. Environ Toxicol Chem. 2005 Aug;24(8):1896-901. doi: 10.1897/04-259r.1. PMID: 16152959.

59. González-Castejón M, Visioli F, Rodriguez-Casado A. Diverse biological activities of dandelion. Nutr Rev. 2012 Sep;70(9):534-47. doi: 10.1111/j.1753-4887.2012.00509.x. Epub 2012 Aug 17. PMID: 22946853.

60. Nathan N. Toxic: Heal Your Body from Mold Toxicity, Lyme Disease, Multiple Chemical Sensitivities, and Chronic Environmental Illness. Victory Belt Publishing, Las Vegas NV. October 9, 2018, p. 73.

61. Henshaw FR, Dewsbury LS, Lim CK, Steiner GZ. The Effects of Cannabinoids on Pro- and Anti-Inflammatory Cytokines: A Systematic Review of *In Vivo* Studies. Cannabis Cannabinoid Res. 2021 Jun;6(3):177-195. doi: 10.1089/can.2020.0105. Epub 2021 Apr 28. PMID: 33998900; PMCID: PMC8266561.

62. Al-Khayri JM, Sahana GR, Nagella P, Joseph BV, Alessa FM, Al-Mssallem MQ. Flavonoids as Potential Anti-Inflammatory Molecules: A Review. Molecules. 2022 May 2;27(9):2901. doi: 10.3390/molecules27092901. PMID: 35566252; PMCID: PMC9100260.

Bibliography

2018 ACVIM Forum Research Abstract Program. Seattle, Washington, June 14 - 15, 2018. J Vet Intern Med. 2018 Nov;32(6):2144-2309. doi: 10.1111/jvim.15319. Epub 2018 Oct 25. PMID: 32744743; PMCID: PMC6272043.

Ajayi AF, Akhigbe RE. Antifertility activity of *Cryptolepis sanguinolenta* leaf ethanolic extract in male rats. J Hum Reprod Sci. 2012 Jan;5(1):43-7.

Alexander W. Integrative Healthcare Symposium: Cancer and Chronic Lyme Disease. P T. 2009 Apr; 34(4): 202–214. PMCID: PMC2697090.

Al-Khayri JM, Sahana GR, Nagella P, Joseph BV, Alessa FM, Al-Mssallem MQ. Flavonoids as Potential Anti-Inflammatory Molecules: A Review. Molecules. 2022 May 2;27(9):2901. doi: 10.3390/molecules27092901. PMID: 35566252; PMCID: PMC9100260.

Álvarez-Martínez FJ, Barrajón-Catalán E, Micol V. Tackling Antibiotic Resistance with Compounds of Natural Origin: A Comprehensive Review.

Biomedicines. 2020 Oct 11;8(10):405. doi: 10.3390/biomedicines8100405. PMID: 33050619; PMCID: PMC7601869.

Aucott JN, Rebman AW, Crowder LA, Kortte KB. Post-treatment Lyme disease syndrome symptomatology and the impact on life functioning: is there something here? Qual Life Res. 2013;22:75–84.

Ayisi, N. K., Appiah-Opong, R., Gyan, B., Bugyei, K., and Ekuban, F. (2011). Plasmodium falciparum: Assessment of Selectivity of Action of Chloroquine, *Alchornea cordifolia, Ficus polita*, and Other Drugs by a Tetrazolium-Based Colorimetric Assay. Malar. Res. Treat 2011, 816250. doi: 10.4061/2011/816250

Banzouzi, J. T., Prado, R., Menan, H., Valentin, A., Roumestan, C., Mallie, M., et al. (2002). In vitro antiplasmodial activity of extracts of *Alchornea cordifolia* and identification of an active constituent: ellagic acid. J. Ethnopharmacol. 81, 399– 401. doi: 10.1016/S0378-8741(02)00121-6

Barthold SW, Hodzic E, Imai DM, Feng S, Yang X, Luft BJ. Ineffectiveness of tigecycline against persistent *Borrelia burgdorferi*. Antimicrob Agents Chemother. 2010;54:643–51.

Basavegowda N, Patra JK, Baek KH. Essential Oils and Mono/bi/tri-Metallic Nanocomposites as Alternative

Sources of Antimicrobial Agents to Combat Multidrug-Resistant Pathogenic Microorganisms: An Overview. Molecules. 2020 Feb 27;25(5):1058. doi: 10.3390/molecules25051058. PMID: 32120930; PMCID: PMC7179174.

Bergsson G, Arnfinnsson J, Steingrímsson Ó, Thormar H. Killing of gram-positive cocci by fatty acids and monoglycerides. APMIS. 2001;109:670–8.

Beshbishy AM, Batiha GE, Yokoyama N, Igarashi I. Ellagic acid microspheres restrict the growth of *Babesia* and *Theileria* in vitro and *Babesia microti* in vivo. Parasit Vectors. 2019 May 28;12(1):269. doi: 10.1186/s13071-019-3520-x. PMID: 31138282; PMCID: PMC6537213.

Bilia AR, Santomauro F, Sacco C, Bergonzi MC, Donato R. Essential Oil of *Artemisia annua* L.: An Extraordinary Component with Numerous Antimicrobial Properties. Evid Based Complement Alternat Med. 2014;2014:159819. doi: 10.1155/2014/159819. Epub 2014 Apr 1. PMID: 24799936; PMCID: PMC3995097.

Boniface, P. K., Ferreira, S. B., and Kaiser, C. R. (2016). Recent trends in phytochemistry, ethnobotany and pharmacological significance of *Alchornea cordifolia* (Schumach. & Thonn.) Muell. Arg. J.

Ethnopharmacol. 191, 216–244. doi: 10.1016/j.jep. 2016.06.021

Borugă O, Jianu C, Mişcă C, Goleţ I, Gruia AT, Horhat FG. *Thymus vulgaris* essential oil: chemical composition and antimicrobial activity. J Med Life. 2014;7:56–60.

Brorson O, Brorson SH. Grapefruit seed extract is a powerful in vitro agent against motile and cystic forms of *Borrelia burgdorferi* sensu lato. Infection. 2007;35:206–8.

Brorson O, Brorson SH. In vitro conversion of *Borrelia burgdorferi* to cystic forms in spinal fluid, and transformation to mobile spirochetes by incubation in BSK-H medium. Infection. 1998;26:144–50.

Buhner, S and Nathan N. Healing Lyme: Natural Healing of Lyme Borreliosis and the Coinfections Chlamydia and Spotted Fever Rickettsiosis, 2nd Edition. Raven Press. Dec 7, 2015.

Buhner, S. Healing Lyme Disease Coinfections: Complementary and Holistic Treatments for *Bartonella* and *Mycoplasma*. Healing Arts Press, Rochester VT. May 5, 2013.

Buhner, S. Herbal Antibiotics, 2nd Edition: Natural Alternatives for Treating Drug-resistant Bacteria. Storey Publishing, North Adams MA. Jul 17, 2012.

Buhner, S. Natural Treatments for Lyme Coinfections: *Anaplasma*, *Babesia*, and *Ehrlichia*. Healing Arts Press, Rochester VT. Feb 22, 2015.

Burt S. Essential oils: their antibacterial properties and potential applications in foods-a review. Int J Food Microbiol. 2004;94:223–53.

Cameron DJ, Johnson L, Maloney EL. Evidence assessments and guideline recommendations in Lyme disease: the clinical management of known tick bites, erythema migrans rashes and persistent disease. Expert Rev Anti-Infect Ther. 2014;12:1103–35.

Centers for Disease Control and Prevention. 2014 Lyme disease website. Available at: http://www.cdc.gov/lyme/. Accessed 13 Sept 2014.

Chaieb K, Hajlaoui H, Zmantar T, Kahla-Nakbi AB, Rouabhia M, Mahdouani K, Bakhrouf A. The chemical composition and biological activity of clove essential oil, *Eugenia caryophyllata* (*Syzigium aromaticum L. Myrtaceae*): a short review. Phytother Res. 2007;21:501–6.

Chen BJ, Fu CS, Li GH, Wang XN, Lou HX, Ren DM, Shen T. Cinnamaldehyde analogues as potential therapeutic agents. Mini Rev Med Chem. 2017;17:33–43.

Chouhan S, Sharma K, Guleria S. Antimicrobial activity of some essential oils-present status and future perspectives. Medicines (Basel). 2017;4:E58.

Cortés-Rojas DF, de Souza CR, Oliveira WP. Clove (*Syzygium aromaticum*): a precious spice. Asian Pac J Trop Biomed. 2014;4:90–6.

Cowan MM. Plant products as antimicrobial agents. Clin Microbiol Rev. 1999;12:564–82.

Cryptolepis (*Cryptolepis sanguinolenta*) — Herbal Monograph (thesunlightexperiment.com). Accessed November 3, 2022.

Cui B, Wang Y, Jin J, Yang Z, Guo R, Li X, Yang L, Li Z. Resveratrol Treats UVB-Induced Photoaging by Anti-MMP Expression, through Anti-Inflammatory, Antioxidant, and Antiapoptotic Properties, and Treats Photoaging by Upregulating VEGF-B Expression. Oxid Med Cell Longev. 2022 Jan 4;2022:6037303. doi: 10.1155/2022/6037303. PMID: 35028009; PMCID: PMC8752231.

Delong AK, Blossom B, Maloney EL, Phillips SE. Antibiotic retreatment of Lyme disease in patients with persistent symptoms: a biostatistical review of randomized, placebo-controlled, clinical trials. Contemp Clin Trials. 2012;33:1132–42.

Desbois AP, Mearns-Spragg A, Smith VJ. A fatty acid from the diatom *Phaeodactylumtricornutum* is antibacterial against diverse bacteria including multi-resistant *Staphylococcusaureus* (MRSA). Mar Biotechnol. 2009;11:45–52.

Desbois AP. Potential applications of antimicrobial fatty acids in medicine, agriculture and other industries. Recent Pat Antiinfect Drug Discov. 2012;7:111–22.

Devi KP, Sakthivel R, Nisha SA, Suganthy N, Pandian SK. Eugenol alters the integrity of cell membrane and acts against the nosocomial pathogen *Proteus mirabilis*. Arch Pharm Res. 2013;36:282–92.

Didehdar M, Chegini Z, Tabaeian SP, Razavi S, Shariati A. *Cinnamomum:* The New Therapeutic Agents for Inhibition of Bacterial and Fungal Biofilm-Associated Infection. Front Cell Infect Microbiol. 2022 Jul 8;12:930624. doi: 10.3389/fcimb.2022.930624. PMID: 35899044; PMCID: PMC9309250.

Draughon FA. Use of botanicals as biopreservatives in foods. Food Technol. 2004;58:20–8.

Ebi, G. C. (2001). Antimicrobial activities of *Alchornea cordifolia*. Fitoterapia 72, 69–72. doi: 10.1016/S0367-326X(00)00254-9

Elfawal MA, Gray O, Dickson-Burke C, Weathers PJ, Rich SM. *Artemisia annua* and artemisinins are ineffective against human *Babesia microti* and six *Candida* sp. Longhua Chin Med. 2021 Jun;4:12. doi: 10.21037/lcm-21-2. PMID: 34316676; PMCID: PMC8312716.

Embers ME, Barthold SW, Borda JT, Bowers L, Doyle L, Hodzic E, Jacobs MB, Hasenkampf NR, Martin DS, Narasimhan S, Phillippi-Falkenstein KM, Purcell JE, Ratterree MS, Philipp MT. Persistence of *Borrelia burgdorferi* in rhesus macaques following antibiotic treatment of disseminated infection. PLoS One. 2012;7:e29914.

Estrada-Peña A, Cevidanes A, Sprong H, Millán J. Pitfalls in Tick and Tick-Borne Pathogens Research, Some Recommendations and a Call for Data Sharing. Pathogens. 2021 Jun 7;10(6):712. doi: 10.3390/pathogens10060712. PMID: 34200175; PMCID: PMC8229135.

Fallon BA, Keilp JG, Corbera KM, Petkova E, Britton CB, Dwyer E, Slavov I, Cheng J, Dobkin J, Nelson DR, Sackeim HA. A randomized, placebo-controlled trial of repeated IV antibiotic therapy for Lyme encephalopathy. Neurology. 2008;70:992–1003.

Fang F, Xie Z, Quan J, Wei X, Wang L, Yang L. Baicalin suppresses Propionibacterium acnes-induced skin inflammation by downregulating the NF-κB/MAPK signaling pathway and inhibiting activation of NLRP3 inflammasome. Braz J Med Biol Res. 2020 Oct 21;53(12):e9949. doi: 10.1590/1414-431X20209949. PMID: 33111746; PMCID: PMC7584154.

Feldlaufer MF, Knox DA, Lusby WR, Shimanuki H. Antimicrobial activity of fatty acids against Bacillus larvae, the causative agent of American foulbrood disease. Apidologie. 1993;24:95–9.

Feng J, Auwaerter PG, Zhang Y. Drug combinations against *Borrelia burgdorferi* persisters in vitro: eradication achieved by using daptomycin, cefoperazone and doxycycline. PLoS One. 2015;10:e0117207.

Feng J, Leone J, Schweig S, Zhang Y. Evaluation of Natural and Botanical Medicines for Activity Against Growing and Non-growing Forms of *B. burgdorferi*. Front Med (Lausanne). 2020 Feb 21;7:6.

doi: 10.3389/fmed.2020.00006. PMID: 32154254; PMCID: PMC7050641.

Feng J, Shi W, Miklossy J, Tauxe GM, McMeniman CJ, Zhang Y. Identification of Essential Oils with Strong Activity against Stationary Phase *Borrelia burgdorferi*. Antibiotics (Basel). 2018 Oct 16;7(4):89. doi: 10.3390/antibiotics7040089. PMID: 30332754; PMCID: PMC6316231.

Feng J, Wang T, Zhang S, Shi W, Zhang Y. An optimized SYBR green I/PI assay for rapid viability assessment and antibiotic susceptibility testing for *Borrelia burgdorferi*. PLoS One. 2014;9:e111809.

Feng J, Zhang S, Shi W, Zhang Y. Ceftriaxone pulse dosing fails to eradicate biofilm-like microcolony *B. Burgdorferi* Persisters which are sterilized by Daptomycin/ doxycycline/cefuroxime without pulse dosing. Front Microbiol. 2016;7:1744–52.

Feng J, Zhang S, Shi W, Zubcevik N, Miklossy J, Zhang Y. Selective Essential Oils from Spice or Culinary Herbs Have High Activity against Stationary Phase and Biofilm *Borrelia burgdorferi*. Front Med (Lausanne). 2017 Oct 11;4:169. doi: 10.3389/fmed.2017.00169. PMID: 29075628; PMCID: PMC5641543.

Feng J, Leone J, Schweig S, and Zhang Y. Evaluation of Natural and Botanical Medicines for Activity Against Growing and Non-growing Forms of *B. burgdorferi*. Front. Med., 21 February 2020 Sec. Infectious Diseases – Surveillance, Prevention and Treatment https://doi.org/10.3389/fmed.2020.00006

Freese E, Shew CW, Galliers E. Function of lipophilic acids as antimicrobial food additives. Nature. 1979;241:321–5.

Friedman M, Buick R, Elliott CT. Antibacterial activities of naturally occurring compounds against antibiotic-resistant *Bacillus cereus* vegetative cells and spores, *Escherichia coli*, and *Staphylococcus aureus*. J Food Prot. 2004;67:1774–8.

Gadila S, Embers ME. Antibiotic Susceptibility of *Bartonella* Grown in Different Culture Conditions. Pathogens . 2021 Jun 8;10(6):718. doi: 10.3390/pathogens10060718. PMID: 34201011 PMCID: PMC8229624.

Ghanim, H., Sia, C. L., Abuaysheh, S., Korzeniewski, K., Patnaik, P., Marumganti, A., et al. (2010). An antiinflammatory and reactive oxygen species suppressive effects of an extract of *Polygonum cuspidatum* containing resveratrol. J. Clin. Endocrinol. Metab. 95, E1–E8. doi: 10.1210/mend.24.7.9998

Goc A, Niedzwiecki A, Rath M. Anti-borreliae efficacy of selected organic oils and fatty acids. BMC Complement Altern Med. 2019 Feb 4;19(1):40. doi: 10.1186/s12906-019-2450-7. PMID: 30717726; PMCID: PMC6360722.

Goc A, Niedzwiecki A, Rath M. Cooperation of Doxycycline with Phytochemicals and Micronutrients Against Active and Persistent Forms of *Borrelia* sp. Int J Biol Sci. 2016 Jul 22;12(9):1093-103. doi: 10.7150/ijbs.16060. PMID: 27570483; PMCID: PMC4997053.

Goc A, Niedzwiecki A, Rath M. In vitro evaluation of antibacterial activity of phytochemicals and micronutrients against *Borrelia burgdorferi* and *Borrelia garinii*. J Appl Microbiol. 2015 Dec;119(6):1561-72. doi: 10.1111/jam.12970. PMID: 26457476; PMCID: PMC4738477.

Goc A, Rath M. The anti-borreliae efficacy of phytochemicals and micronutrients: an update. Ther Adv Infect Dis. 2016 Jun;3(3-4):75-82. doi: 10.1177/ 2049936116655502. Epub 2016 Jul 4. PMID: 27536352; PMCID: PMC4971593.

González-Castejón M, Visioli F, Rodriguez-Casado A. Diverse biological activities of dandelion. Nutr Rev. 2012 Sep;70(9):534-47. doi: 10.1111/j.1753-4887. 2012.00509.x. Epub 2012 Aug 17. PMID: 22946853.

Greenway DLA, Dyke KGH. Mechanism of the inhibitory action of linoleic acid on the growth of *Staphylococcus aureus*. J Gen Microbiol. 1979;115:233–45.

Heath RJ, White SW, Rock CO. Lipid biosynthesis as a target for antibacterial agents. Prog Lipid Res. 2001;40:467–97.

Henshaw FR, Dewsbury LS, Lim CK, Steiner GZ. The Effects of Cannabinoids on Pro- and Anti-Inflammatory Cytokines: A Systematic Review of *In Vivo* Studies. Cannabis Cannabinoid Res. 2021 Jun;6(3):177-195. doi: 10.1089/can.2020.0105. Epub 2021 Apr 28. PMID: 33998900; PMCID: PMC8266561.

Hirooka T, Nagase H, Uchida K, Hiroshige Y, Ehara Y, Nishikawa J, Nishihara T, Miyamoto K, Hirata Z. Biodegradation of bisphenol A and disappearance of its estrogenic activity by the green alga *Chlorella fusca* var. vacuolata. Environ Toxicol Chem. 2005 Aug;24(8):1896-901. doi: 10.1897/04-259r.1. PMID: 16152959.

Ho KV, Schreiber KL, Vu DC, Rottinghaus SM, Jackson DE, Brown CR, Lei Z, Sumner LW, Coggeshall MV, Lin CH. Black Walnut (*Juglans nigra*) Extracts Inhibit Proinflammatory Cytokine Production From Lipopolysaccharide-Stimulated Human Promonocytic Cell Line U-937. Front Pharmacol. 2019 Sep 19;

10:1059. doi: 10.3389/fphar.2019.01059. PMID: 31607915; PMCID: PMC6761373.

Horowitz RI, Freeman PR. Precision Medicine: The Role of the MSIDS Model in Defining, Diagnosing, and Treating Chronic Lyme Disease/Post Treatment Lyme Disease Syndrome and Other Chronic Illness: Part 2. Healthcare (Basel). 2018 Nov 5;6(4):129. doi: 10.3390/healthcare6040129. PMID: 30400667; PMCID: PMC6316761.

https://thenaturopathicherbalist.com/herbs/i-l/juglans-nigra-black-walnut/ Marisa Marciano. Accessed November 3, 2022.

https://woodlandessence.com/products/black-walnut-liquid-extract. Accessed November 3, 2022.

https://www.cdc.gov/malaria/diagnosis_treatment/discontinuation_artesunate.html.

https://www.cdc.gov/malaria/new_info/2020/artesunate_approval.html. Accessed, November 3, 2022.

https://www.rxlist.com/artesunate-drug.htm. Accessed November 3, 2022

Hubálek Z, Rudolf I. Systematic Survey of Zoonotic and Sapronotic Microbial Agents. Microbial Zoonoses and Sapronoses. 2010 Nov 10 : 129–297. Published online 2010 Nov 10. doi: 10.1007/978-90-481-9657-9_8. PMCID: PMC7119992.

Jansen FH. The pharmaceutical death-ride of dihydroartemisinin. Malar J. 2010 Jul 22;9:212. doi: 10.1186/1475-2875-9-212. PMID: 20649950; PMCID: PMC2916014.

Jayaprakasha GK, Rao LJ. Chemistry, biogenesis, and biological activities of *Cinnamomum zeylanicum*. Crit Rev Food Sci Nutr. 2011;51:547–62.

Jiang BG, Jia N, Jiang JF, Zheng YC, Chu YL, Jiang RR, Wang YW, Liu HB, Wei R, Zhang WH, Li Y, Xu XW, Ye JL, Yao NN, Liu XJ, Huo QB, Sun Y, Song JL, Liu W, Cao WC. *Borrelia miyamotoi* Infections in Humans and Ticks, Northeastern China. Emerg Infect Dis. 2018 Feb;24(2):236-241. doi: 10.3201/eid2402.160378. PMID: 29350133; PMCID: PMC5782893.

Juteau F, Masotti V, Bessière JM, Dherbomez M, Viano J. Antibacterial and antioxidant activities of *Artemisia annua* essential oil. Fitoterapia. 2002 Oct;73(6): 532-5. doi: 10.1016/s0367-326x(02)00175-2. PMID: 12385883.

Kabara JJ, Swieczkowski DM, Conley AJ, Truant JP. Fatty acids and derivatives as antimicrobial agents. Antimicrob Agents Chemother. 1972;2:23–8.

Kabara JJ, Vrable R. Antimicrobial lipids: natural and synthetic fatty acids and monoglycerides. Lipids. 1977;12:753–9.

Karbach J, Ebenezer S, Warnke PH, Behrens E, Al-Nawas B. Antimicrobial effect of Australian antibacterial essential oils as alternative to common antiseptic solutions against clinically relevant oral pathogens. Clin Lab. 2015;61:616–8.

Kuchta K, Cameron S. Tradition to Pathogenesis: A Novel Hypothesis for Elucidating the Pathogenesis of Diseases Based on the Traditional Use of Medicinal Plants. Front Pharmacol. 2021 Oct 25;12:705077. doi: 10.3389/fphar.2021.705077. PMID: 34759818; PMCID: PMC8572966.

Laldinsangi C. The therapeutic potential of *Houttuynia cordata*: A current review. Heliyon. 2022 Aug 24;8(8):e10386. doi: 10.1016/j.heliyon.2022.e10386. PMID: 36061012; PMCID: PMC9433674.

Lamikanra, A., Ogundaini, A. O., and Ogungbamila, F. O. (1990). Antibacterial Constituents of *Alchornea-Cordifolia* Leaves. Phytother. Res. 4, 198–200. doi: 10.1002/ptr.2650040508

Lee CW, Kim SC, Kwak TW, Lee JR, Jo MJ, Ahn Y-T, Kim JM, An WG. Anti-Inflammatory Effects of Bangpungtongsung-San, a Traditional Herbal

Prescription. Evid Based Complement Alternat Med. 2012; 2012: 892943. Published online 2012 Jul 29. doi: 10.1155/2012/892943. PMCID: PMC3414209.

Leyva Salas M, Mounier J, Valence F, Coton M, Thierry A, Coton E. Antifungal microbial agents for food biopreservation-a review. Microorganisms. 2017;5:E37.

Liebold T, Straubinger RK, Rauwald HW. Growth inhibiting activity of lipophilic extracts from *Dipsacus sylvestris Huds*. roots against *Borrelia burgdorferi* s. s. in vitro. Pharmazie. 2011 Aug;66(8):628-30. PMID: 21901989.

Loewen PS, Marra CA, Marra F. Systematic review of the treatment of early Lyme disease. Drugs. 1999; 57:157–73.

Lu M, Dai T, Murray CK, Wu MX. Bactericidal Property of Oregano Oil Against Multidrug-Resistant Clinical Isolates. Front Microbiol. 2018 Oct 5;9:2329. doi: 10.3389/fmicb.2018.02329. Erratum in: Front Microbiol. 2021 Jul 12;12:713573. PMID: 30344513; PMCID: PMC6182053.

Ma X, Shi W, Zhang Y. Essential Oils with High Activity against Stationary Phase *Bartonella henselae*. Antibiotics (Basel). 2019 Nov 30;8(4):246. doi: 10.3390/

antibiotics8040246. PMID: 31801196; PMCID: PMC6963529.

Ma, Xiao; Leone, Jacob; Schweig, Sunjya; Zhang, Ying. Botanical Medicines With Activity Against Stationary Phase Bartonella henselae. Infectious Microbes & Diseases 3(3):p 158-167, September 2021. doi: 10.1097/IM9.0000000000000069

Maitland J, Fleming SA. Organic Chemistry. United Kingdom: W. W. Norton & Co Inc (Np); 1998.

Manga, H. M., Brkic, D., Marie, D. E., and Quetin-Leclercq, J. (2004). In vivo antiinflammatory activity of *Alchornea cordifolia* (Schumach. Thonn.) Mull. Arg. (Euphorbiaceae). J. Ethnopharmacol. 92, 209–214. doi: 10.1016/ j.jep.2004.02.019

Martin KW, Ernst E. Herbal medicines for treatment of bacterial infections: a review of controlled clinical trials. J Antimicrob Chemother. 2003;51:241–6.

Marzec NS, Nelson C, Waldron PR, Blackburn BG, Hosain S, Greenhow T, Green GM, Lomen-Hoerth C, Golden M, Mead PS. Serious Bacterial Infections Acquired During Treatment of Patients Given a Diagnosis of Chronic Lyme Disease - United States. MMWR Morb Mortal Wkly Rep. 2017 Jun 16;66(23):607-609. doi: 10.15585/mmwr.mm6623a3. PMID: 28617768; PMCID: PMC5657841.

Mayaud L, Carricajo A, Zhiri A, Aubert G. Comparison of bacteriostatic and bactericidal activity of 13 essential oils against strains with varying sensitivity to antibiotics. Lett Appl Microbiol. 2008;47:167–73.

McHale D, Laurie WA, Woof MA. Composition of west Indian bay oils. Food Chem. 1977;2:19–25.

Melo AD, Amaral AF, Schaefer G, Luciano FB, de Andrade C, Costa LB, Rostagno MH. Antimicrobial effect against different bacterial strains and bacterial adaptation to essential oils used as feed additives. Can J Microbiol. 2015;61:263–71.

Mesia, G. K., Tona, G. L., Nanga, T. H., Cimanga, R. K., Apers, S., Cos, P., et al. (2008). Antiprotozoal and cytotoxic screening of 45 plant extracts from Democratic Republic of Congo. J. Ethnopharmacol. 115, 409–415. doi: 10.1016/j.jep.2007.10.028

Morrison KC, Hergenrother PJ. Natural products as starting points for the synthesis of complex and diverse compounds. Nat Prod Rep. 2014;31:6–14.

Murgia R, Cinco M. Induction of cystic forms by different stress conditions in *Borrelia burgdorferi*. APMIS. 2004;112:57–62.

Mustofa, A., Benoit-Vical, F., Pelissier, Y., Kone-Bamba, D., and Mallie, M. (2000). Antiplasmodial activity of plant extracts used-in west African traditional medicine. J. Ethnopharmacol. 73, 145–151. doi: 10.1016/S0378-8741(00) 00296-8

Nabavi SF, Di Lorenzo A, Izadi M, Sobarzo-Sánchez E, Daglia M, Nabavi SM. Antibacterial effects of cinnamon: from farm to food, cosmetic and pharmaceutical industries. Nutrients. 2015;7:7729–48.

Nair A, Mallya R, Suvarna V, Khan TA, Momin M, Omri A. Nanoparticles-Attractive Carriers of Antimicrobial Essential Oils. Antibiotics (Basel). 2022 Jan 14;11(1):108. doi: 10.3390/antibiotics11010108. PMID: 35052985; PMCID: PMC8773333.

Nathan N. Toxic: Heal Your Body from Mold Toxicity, Lyme Disease, Multiple Chemical Sensitivities, and Chronic Environmental Illness. Victory Belt Publishing, Las Vegas NV. October 9, 2018.

Nazzaro F, Fratianni F, De Martino L, Coppola R, De Feo V. Effect of essential oils on pathogenic bacteria. Pharmaceuticals (Basel). 2013;6:1451–74.

Oguntomole O, Nwaeze U, Eremeeva ME. Tick-, Flea-, and Louse-Borne Diseases of Public Health and Veterinary Significance in Nigeria. Trop Med Infect Dis. 2018 Jan 3;3(1):3. doi: 10.3390/tropicalmed3010003. PMID: 30274402; PMCID: PMC6136614.

Okhuarobo A, Faludun JE, Erharuyi O, Imieje V, Falodun A, Langer P. Harnessing the medicinal properties of *Andrographis paniculata* for diseases and beyond: a review of its phytochemistry and pharmacology. Asian Pac J Trop Dis. 2014 Jun; 4(3): 213–222. doi: 10.1016/S2222-1808(14)60509-0

Ooi LS, Li Y, Kam SL, Wang H, Wong EY, Ooi VE. Antimicrobial activities of cinnamon oil and cinnamaldehyde from the Chinese medicinal herb *Cinnamomum cassia Blume*. Am J Chin Med. 2006;34:511–22.

Pang J, Dong W, Li Y, Xia X, Liu Z, Hao H, Jiang L, Liu Y. Purification of *Houttuynia cordata Thunb*. Essential Oil Using Macroporous Resin Followed by Microemulsion Encapsulation to Improve Its Safety and Antiviral Activity. Molecules. 2017 Feb 15;22(2):293. doi: 10.3390/molecules22020293. PMID: 28212296; PMCID: PMC6155675.

Patterson SL, Jafri K, Narvid JA, Margaretten M. A Young Woman With Sudden Urinary Retention and Sensory Deficits. Arthritis Care Res (Hoboken). 2018 Apr;70(4):635-642. doi: 10.1002/acr.23473. Epub 2018 Feb 18. PMID: 29125903; PMCID: PMC5876077.

Pisoschi AM, Pop A, Georgescu C, Turcuş V, Olah NK. Mathe EAn overview of natural antimicrobials role in food. Eur J Med Chem. 2018;143:922–35.

Pizzorno JF, Murray MT. Textbook of Natural Medicine - 2-volume set 5th Edition. Churchill Livingstone. July 13, 2020.

Price RN, Douglas NM. Artemisinin combination therapy for malaria: beyond good efficacy. Clin Infect Dis.2009Dec1;49(11):1638-40.doi:10.1086/647947. PMID: 19877970; PMCID: PMC4627500.

Rawls, B. The Cellular Wellness Solution: Tap Into Your Full Health Potential with the Science-Backed Power of Herbs. June 18, 2022, First Do No Harm Publishing, Raleigh NC.

Rudenko N, Golovchenko M, Kybicova K, Vancova M. Metamorphoses of Lyme disease spirochetes: phenomenon of *Borrelia* persisters. Parasit Vectors. 2019 May 16;12(1):237. doi: 10.1186/s13071-019-3495-7. PMID: 31097026; PMCID: PMC6521364.

Saar-Reismaa P, Bragina O, Kuhtinskaja M, Reile I, Laanet PR, Kulp M, Vaher M. Extraction and Fractionation of Bioactives from *Dipsacus fullonum* L. Leaves and Evaluation of Their Anti-*Borrelia* Activity. Pharmaceuticals (Basel). 2022 Jan 12;15(1):87.

doi: 10.3390/ph15010087. PMID: 35056144; PMCID: PMC8779505.

Sandborn WJ, Targan SR, Byers VS, Rutty DA, Mu H, Zhang X, Tang T. *Andrographis paniculata* extract (HMPL-004) for active ulcerative colitis. Am J Gastroenterol. 2013 Jan;108(1):90-8. doi: 10.1038/ajg.2012.340. Epub 2012 Oct 9. PMID: 23044768; PMCID: PMC3538174.

Sapi E, Balasubramanian K, Poruri A, Maghsoudlou JS, Socarras KM, Timmaraju AV, Filush KR, Gupta K, Shaikh S, Theophilus PA, Luecke DF, MacDonald A, Zelger B. Evidence of in vivo existence of *Borrelia* biofilm in Borrelial Lymphocytomas. Eur J Microbiol Immunol (Bp). 2016;6:9–24.

Sapi E, Bastian SL, Mpoy CM, Scott S, Rattelle A, Pabbati N, Poruri A, Burugu D, Theophilus PA, Pham TV, Datar A, Dhaliwal NK, MacDonald A, Rossi MJ, Sinha SK, Luecke DF. Characterization of biofilm formation by *Borrelia burgdorferi* in vitro. PLoS One. 2012;7:e48277.

Sapi E, Kaur N, Anyanwu S, Luecke DF, Datar A, Patel S, Rossi M, Stricker RB. Evaluation of in-vitro antibiotic susceptibility of different morphological forms of *Borrelia burgdorferi*. Infect Drug Resist. 2011;4:97–113.

Schaller J. A Laboratory Guide to Human *Babesia* Hematology Forms. Hope Academic Press, Tampa FL. Sep 15, 2008.

Schaller, J. Artemisinin, Artesunate, Artemisinic Acid and Other Derivatives of *Artemisia* Used for Malaria, *Babesia* and Cancer. Hope Academic Press, Tampa FL. October 13, 2006.

Schaller J. The Health Care Professional's Guide to the Treatment and Diagnosis of Human Babesiosis: An Extensive Review of New Human *Babesia* Species and Advanced Treatments. Hope Academic Press, Tampa FL. Oct 16, 2006.

Schaller J. What You May Not Know About *Bartonella, Babesia*, Lyme Disease and Other Tick & Flea-borne Infections: Improving Treatment Speed, Recovery & Patient Satisfaction. International University Infectious Disease Press, Naples FL. Feb 8, 2012.

Schaller J, Mountjoy K. Checklists for *Bartonella, Babesia* and Lyme Disease. International Academic Infection Research Press, Dec 27, 2011.

Schaller J, Mountjoy K. Combating Biofilms. International Infectious Disease Press. Naples FL. April 11, 2014.

Schauenstein E. Autoxidation of polyunsaturated esters in water: chemical structure and biological activity of the products. J Lipid Res. 1967;8:417–28.

Scott JD, McGoey E, Pesapane RR. Tick-Borne Pathogens *Anaplasma phagocytophilum, Babesia odocoilei*, and *Borrelia burgdorferi* Sensu Lato in Blacklegged Ticks Widespread across Eastern Canada. 2022 Oct 27; 3(10): 1249-1256. doi: 10.37871/jbres1586, Article ID: JBRES1586, Available at: https://www.jelsciences.com/articles/jbres1586.pdf

Seidel V, Taylor PW. In vitro activity of extracts and constituents of Pelagonium against rapidly growing mycobacteria. Int J Antimicrob Agents. 2004;23:613–9.

Shan, B., Cai, Y. Z., Brooks, J. D., and Corke, H. (2008). Antibacterial properties of *Polygonum cuspidatum* roots and their major bioactive constituents. Food Chem. 109, 530–537. doi: 10.1016/j.foodchem.2007.12.064

Shapiro ED. Lyme disease. N Engl J Med. 2014; 370:1724–31.

Sharma B, Brown AV, Matluck NE, Hu LT, Lewis K. *Borrelia burgdorferi*, the causative agent of

Lyme disease, forms drug-tolerant persister cells. Antimicrob Agents Chemother. 2015;59:4616–24.

Singh O, Khanam Z, Misra N, Srivastava MK. Chamomile (*Matricaria chamomilla L.*): An overview. Appl Microbiol Biotechnol. 2010;85:1629–42.

Smith-Palmer A, Stewart J, Fyfe L. Antimicrobial properties of plant essential oils and essences against five important food-borne pathogens. Lett Appl Microbiol. 1998;26:118–22.

Straubinger RK, Summers BA, Chang YF, Appel MJ. Persistence of *Borrelia burgdorferi* in experimentally infected dogs after antibiotic treatment. J Clin Microbiol. 1997;35:111–6.

Sun CQ, O'Connor CJ, Roberton AM. Antibacterial actions of fatty acids and monoglycerides against *helicobacter pylori*. FEMS Immunol Med Microbiol. 2003;36:9–17.

Suriyo T, Pholphana N, Ungtrakul T, Rangkadilok N, Panomvana D, Thiantanawat A, Pongpun W, Satayavivad J. Clinical Parameters following Multiple Oral Dose Administration of a Standardized *Andrographis paniculata* Capsule in Healthy Thai Subjects. Planta Med. 2017 Jun;83(9):778-789. doi: 10.1055/s-0043-104382. Epub 2017 Mar 1. PMID: 28249303.

Tanaka M, Kishimoto Y, Sasaki M, Sato A, Kamiya T, Kondo K, Iida K. *Terminalia bellirica* (Gaertn.) Roxb. Extract and Gallic Acid Attenuate LPS-Induced Inflammation and Oxidative Stress via MAPK/NF-κB and Akt/AMPK/Nrf2 Pathways. Oxid Med Cell Longev. 2018 Nov 8;2018:9364364. doi: 10.1155/2018/9364364. PMID: 30533177; PMCID: PMC6250009.

Tang T, Targan SR, Li ZS, Xu C, Byers VS, Sandborn WJ. Randomised clinical trial: herbal extract HMPL-004 in active ulcerative colitis - a double-blind comparison with sustained release mesalazine. Aliment Pharmacol Ther. 2011 Jan;33(2):194-202. doi: 10.1111/j.1365-2036.2010.04515.x. Epub 2010 Nov 30. PMID: 21114791.

Theophilus PA, Victoria MJ, Socarras KM, Filush KR, Gupta K, Luecke DF, Sapi E. Effectiveness of stevia Rebaudiana whole leaf extract against the various morphological forms of *Borrelia Burgdorferi* in vitro. Eur J Microbiol Immunol. (Bp). 2015;5:268–80.

Thormar H, Hilmarsson H. The role of microbicidal lipids in host defense against pathogens and their potential as therapeutic agents. Chem Phys Lipids. 2007;150:1–11.

Tisserand R, Young R. Essential Oil Safety. United Kingdom: Churchill Livingstone Elsevier; 2013.

Trinh NT, Dumas E, Thanh ML, Degraeve P, Ben Amara C, Gharsallaoui A, Oulahal N. Effect of a Vietnamese *Cinnamomum cassia* essential oil and its major component trans-cinnamaldehyde on the cell viability, membrane integrity, membrane fluidity, and proton motive force of *Listeria innocua*. Can J Microbiol. 2015;61:263–71.

Vojdani A, Erde J. Regulatory T Cells, a Potent Immunoregulatory Target for CAM Researchers: Modulating Tumor Immunity, Autoimmunity and Alloreactive Immunity (III). Evid Based Complement Alternat Med. 2006 Sep; 3(3): 309–316. Published online 2006 Jul 5. doi: 10.1093/ecam/nel047. PMCID: PMC1513145.

Vojdani A, Hebroni F, Raphael Y, Erde J, Raxlen B. Novel Diagnosis of Lyme Disease: Potential for CAM Intervention. Evid Based Complement Alternat Med. 2009 Sep; 6(3): 283–295. Published online 2007 Oct 15. doi: 10.1093/ecam/nem138. PMCID: PMC2722197.

Wang M, Firrman J, Zhang L, Arango-Argoty G, Tomasula P, Liu L, Xiao W, Yam K. Apigenin Impacts the Growth of the Gut Microbiota and Alters the Gene Expression of Enterococcus. Molecules. 2017 Aug 3;22(8):1292. doi: 10.3390/molecules22081292. PMID: 28771188; PMCID: PMC6152273.

Willcox M, Bodeke G, Rasoanalvo P, Addae-Kyereme J (eds). Traditional Medicinal Plants and Malaria (Traditional Herbal Medicines for Modern Times) 1st Edition. CRC Press. 2004

Wińska K, Mączka W, Łyczko J, Grabarczyk M, Czubaszek A, Szumny A. Essential Oils as Antimicrobial Agents-Myth or Real Alternative? Molecules. 2019 Jun 5;24(11):2130. doi: 10.3390/molecules24112130. PMID: 31195752; PMCID: PMC6612361.

Xue C, Chen Y, Hu DN, Iacob C, Lu C, Huang Z. Chrysin induces cell apoptosis in human uveal melanoma cells via intrinsic apoptosis. Oncol Lett. 2016 Dec;12(6):4813-4820. doi: 10.3892/ol.2016.5251. Epub 2016 Oct 13. PMID: 28105189; PMCID: PMC5228444.

Yousef RT, Tawil GG. Antimicrobial activity of volatile oils. Pharmazie. 1980;35:698–701.

Zalegh I, Akssira M, Bourhia M, Mellouki F, Rhallabi N, Salamatullah AM, Alkaltham MS, Khalil Alyahya H, Mhand RA. A Review on *Cistus* sp.: Phytochemical and Antimicrobial Activities. Plants (Basel). 2021 Jun 15;10(6):1214. doi: 10.3390/plants10061214. PMID: 34203720; PMCID: PMC8232106.

Zhang H, Li C, Kwok ST, Zhang QW, Chan SW. A Review of the Pharmacological Effects of the Dried

Root of *Polygonum cuspidatum* (Hu Zhang) and Its Constituents. Evid Based Complement Alternat Med. 2013;2013:208349. doi: 10.1155/2013/208349. Epub 2013 Sep 30. PMID: 24194779; PMCID: PMC3806114. (Hidawi)

Zhang H, Li S, Si Y, Xu H. Andrographolide and its derivatives: Current achievements and future perspectives. Eur J Med Chem. 2021 Nov 15;224: 113710. doi: 10.1016/j.ejmech.2021.113710. Epub 2021 Jul 20. PMID: 34315039.

Zhang Q, Zhao JJ, Xu J, Feng F, Qu W. Medicinal uses, phytochemistry and pharmacology of the genus *Uncaria*. J Ethnopharmacol. 2015 Sep 15;173:48-80. doi: 10.1016/j.jep.2015.06.011. Epub 2015 Jun 17. PMID: 26091967.

Zhang QC, Zhang Y. Lyme Disease and Modern Chinese Medicine. Sino-Med research Institute, New York, NY. March 1, 2006.

Zhang Y, Alvarez-Manzo H, Leone J, Schweig S and Zhang Y. (2021)Botanical Medicines *Cryptolepis sanguinolenta, Artemisia annua, Scutellaria baicalensis, Polygonumcuspidatum*, and *Alchornea cordifolia* Demonstrate Inhibitory Activity Against *Babesia duncani*. Front. Cell. Infect. Microbiol. 11:624745. doi: 10.3389/fcimb.2021.624745

Zhang Y, Bai C, Shi W, Alvarez-Manzo H, Zhang Y. Identification of Essential Oils Including Garlic Oil and Black Pepper Oil with High Activity against *Babesia duncani*. Pathogens. 2020 Jun 12;9(6):466. doi: 10.3390/pathogens9060466. PMID: 32545549; PMCID: PMC7350376.

Zhou YX, Zhang H, Peng C. Puerarin: a review of pharmacological effects. Phytother Res. 2014 Jul;28(7):961-75. doi: 10.1002/ptr.5083. Epub 2013 Dec 13. PMID: 24339367.